The Definitive Air Fryer Cooking Guide

Incredible Air Fryer Recipes For Everyone

Ellie Sloan

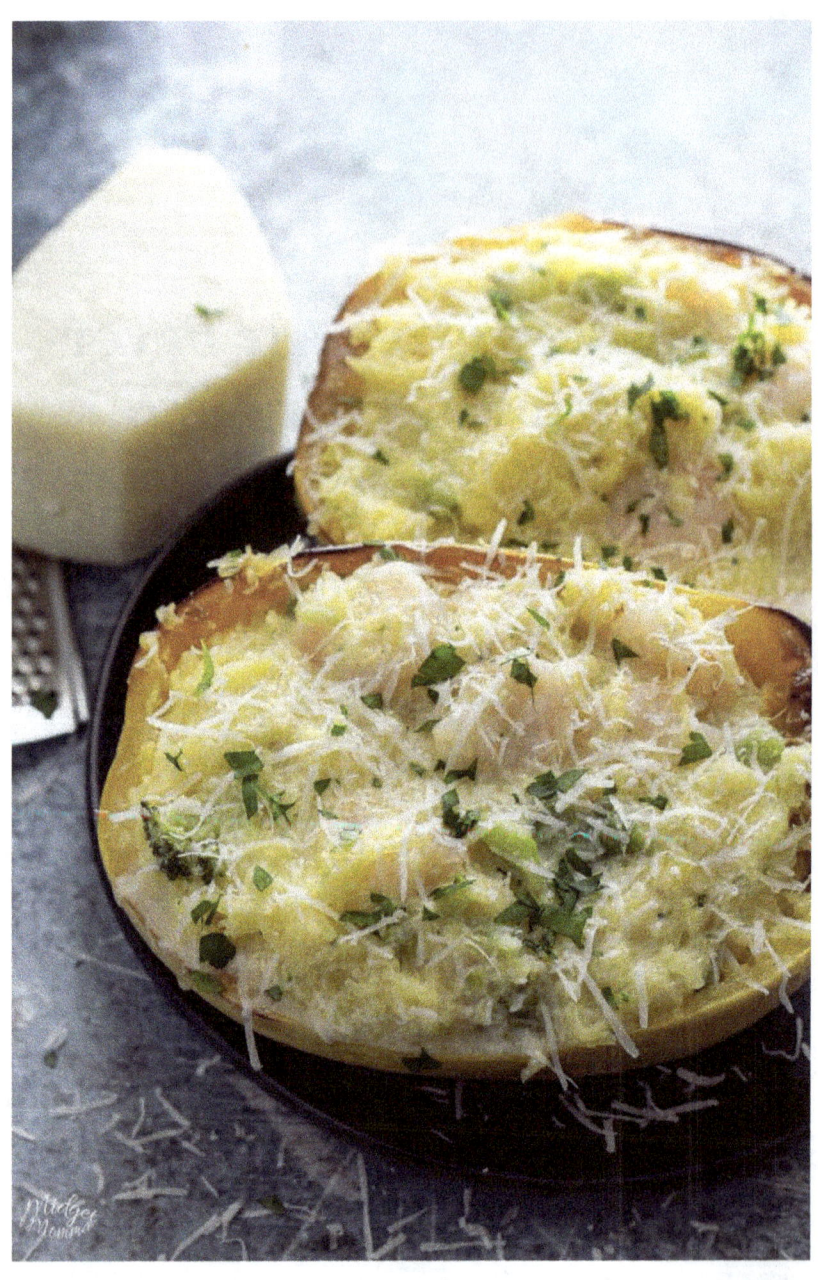

© **Copyright 2020 - All rights reserved.**

The content contained within this book may not be reproduced, duplicated or transmitted without direct written permission from the author or the publisher.

Under no circumstances will any blame or legal responsibility be held against the publisher, or author, for any damages, reparation, or monetary loss due to the information contained within this book. Either directly or indirectly.

Legal Notice:

This book is copyright protected. This book is only for personal use. You cannot amend, distribute, sell, use, quote or paraphrase any part, or the content within this book, without the consent of the author or publisher.

Disclaimer Notice:

Please note the information contained within this document is for educational and entertainment purposes only. All effort has been executed to present accurate, up to date, and reliable, complete information. No warranties of any kind are declared or implied. Readers acknowledge that the author is not engaging in the rendering of legal, financial, medical or professional advice. The content within this book has been derived from various sources. Please consult a licensed professional before attempting any techniques outlined in this book.

By reading this document, the reader agrees that under no circumstances is the author responsible for any losses, direct or indirect, which are incurred as a result of the use of information contained within this document, including, but not limited to, — errors, omissions, or inaccuracies.

Table of contents

Burrata-Stuffed Tomatoes 7
Broccoli with Parmesan Cheese 9
Caramelized Broccoli 11
Brussels Sprouts with Balsamic Oil 13
Spiced Butternut Squash 15
Garlic Thyme Mushrooms 17
Zucchini Parmesan Chips 19
Jicama Fries 21
Lemon bell peppers 23
Cauliflower pizza crust 25
Savoy cabbage and tomatoes 27
Cauliflower steak 29
Tomato, avocado and green beans 31
Dill and garlic green beans 33
Eggplant stacks 35
Air Fried Spaghetti Squash 37
Beets and Blue Cheese Salad 39
Broccoli Salad 41
Roasted Brussels Sprouts with Tomatoes 43
Cheesy Brussels Sprouts 45
Sweet Baby Carrots Dish 47
Seasoned Leeks 49

Crispy Potatoes and Parsley	51
Garlic Tomatoes	53
Easy Green Beans and Potatoes	55
Green Beans and Tomatoes	57
Flavored Asparagus	59
Spaghetti Squash Tots	61
Cinnamon Butternut Squash Fries	63
Cheesy Roasted Sweet Potatoes	65
Salty Lemon Artichokes	67
Asparagus & Parmesan	69
Corn on Cobs	72
Onion Green Beans	74
Dill Mashed Potato	76
Cream Potato	78
Chard with Cheddar	80
Chili Squash Wedges	82
Honey Carrots with Greens	84
South Asian Cauliflower Fritters	86
Supreme Air-Fried Tofu	88
Lemon Bars	90
Coconut Donuts	92
Blueberry Cream	94
Blackberry Chia Jam	96
Mixed Berries Cream	98

Apple Chips 100

Sweetened Plantains 102

Roasted Bananas 104

Pear Crisp 106

Burrata-Stuffed Tomatoes

Preparation Time: 5 minutes

Cooking Time: 5 minutes

Servings: 4

Ingredients:

- 4 medium tomatoes
- ½ tsp. fine sea salt
- 4 (2 oz.) Burrata balls
- Fresh basil leaves, for garnish
- Extra-virgin olive oil, for drizzling

Directions:

1. Preheat the Air Fryer to 300°F.
2. Scoop out the tomato seeds and membranes using a melon baller or spoon. Sprinkle the insides of the tomatoes with the salt. Stuff each tomato with a ball of Burrata.

3. Put it in the fryer and cook for 5 minutes, or until the cheese has softened.
4. Garnish with olive oil and basil leaves. Serve warm.

Nutrition:

Calories 108

Fat 7g

Carbs 5g

Protein 6g

Broccoli with Parmesan Cheese

Preparation Time: 5 minutes

Cooking Time: 5 minutes

Servings: 4

Ingredients:

- 1 lb. broccoli florets
- 2 tsp.s minced garlic
- 2 tbsp. olive oil
- ¼ cup grated or shaved Parmesan cheese

Directions

1. Preheat the Air Fryer to 360°F. In a bowl, mix together the broccoli florets, garlic, olive oil, and Parmesan cheese.
2. Place the broccoli in the Air Fryer basket in a single layer and set the timer and steam for 4 minutes.

Nutrition:

Calories 130

Fat 3g

Carbs 5g

Protein 4g

Caramelized Broccoli

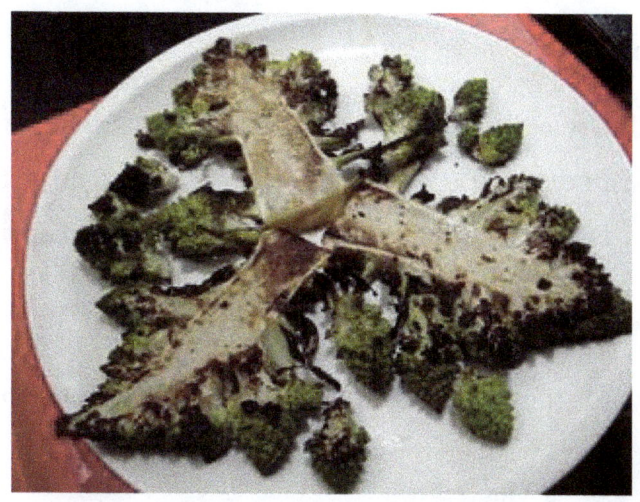

Preparation Time: 5 minutes

Cooking Time: 10 minutes

Servings: 4

Ingredients:

- 4 cups broccoli florets
- 3 tbsp. melted ghee or butter-flavored coconut oil
- 1½ tsp.s fine sea salt or smoked salt

- Mayonnaise, for serving (optional; omit for egg-free)

Directions

1. Grease the basket with avocado oil. Preheat the Air Fryer to 400°F. Place the broccoli in a large bowl. Drizzle it with the ghee, toss to coat, and sprinkle it with the salt.
2. Transfer the broccoli to the Air Fryer basket and cook for 8 minutes, or until tender and crisp on the edges.

Nutrition:

Calories 120

Fat 2g

Carbs 4g

Protein 3g

Brussels Sprouts with Balsamic Oil

Preparation Time: 5 minutes

Cooking Time: 15 minutes

Servings: 4

Ingredients:

- ¼ tsp. salt
- 1 tbsp. balsamic vinegar
- 2cups Brussels sprouts, halved
- 3tbsp. olive oil

Directions:

1. Preheat the Air Fryer for 5 minutes. Mix all ingredients in a bowl until the zucchini fries are well coated.
2. Place in the Air Fryer basket. Close and cook for 15 minutes for 350°F.

Nutrition:

Calories 82

Fat 6.8g

Carbs 2g

Protein 1.5g

Spiced Butternut Squash

Preparation Time: 10 minutes

Cooking Time: 15 minutes

Servings: 4

Ingredients:

- 4 cups 1-inch-cubed butternut squash
- 2 tbsp. vegetable oil
- 1 to 2 tbsp. brown sugar
- 1 tsp. Chinese five-spice powder

Directions:

1. In a bowl, combine the oil, sugar, squash, and five-spice powder. Toss to coat.
2. Place the squash in the Air Fryer basket.
3. Set the Air Fryer to 400°F for 15 minutes or until tender.

Nutrition:

Calories 160

Fat 5g

Carbs 9g

Protein 6g

Garlic Thyme Mushrooms

Preparation Time: 5 minutes

Cooking Time: 10 minutes

Servings: 4

Ingredients:

- 3 tbsp. unsalted butter, melted
- 1 (8 oz.) package button mushrooms, sliced
- 2 cloves garlic, minced
- 3 sprigs fresh thyme leaves
- ½ tsp. fine sea salt

Directions:

1. Grease the basket with avocado oil. Preheat the Air Fryer to 400°F.
2. Place all the ingredients in a medium-sized bowl. Use a spoon or your hands to coat the mushroom slices.
3. Put the mushrooms in the basket in one layer; work in batches if necessary. Cook for 10 minutes, or until

slightly crispy and brown. Garnish with thyme sprigs before serving.
4. Reheat in a warmed up 350°F Air Fryer for 5 minutes, or until heated through.

Nutrition:

Calories 82

Fat 9g

Carbs 1g

Protein 1g

Zucchini Parmesan Chips

Preparation Time: 10 minutes

Cooking Time: 10 minutes

Servings: 10

Ingredients:

- ½ tsp. paprika
- ½ C. grated parmesan cheese
- ½ C. Italian breadcrumbs
- 1 lightly beaten egg
- 2 thinly sliced zucchinis

Directions:

1. Use a very sharp knife or mandolin slicer to slice zucchini as thinly as you can. Pat off extra moisture. Beat egg with a pinch of pepper and salt and a bit of water.

2. Combine paprika, cheese, and breadcrumbs in a bowl. Dip slices of zucchini into the egg mixture and then into breadcrumb mixture. Press gently to coat.
3. With olive oil cooking spray, mist coated zucchini slices. Place into your Air Fryer in a single layer. Set temperature to 350°F, and set time to 8 minutes. Sprinkle with salt and serve with salsa.

Nutrition:

Calories 130

Fat 2g

Carbs 5g

Protein 3g

Jicama Fries

Preparation Time: 10 minutes

Cooking Time: 5 minutes

Servings: 4

Ingredients:

- 1 tbsp. dried thyme
- ¾ C. arrowroot flour
- ½ large Jicama
- Eggs

Directions:

1. Sliced jicama into fries.
2. Whisk eggs together and pour over fries. Toss to coat.
3. Mix a pinch of salt, thyme, and arrowroot flour together. Toss egg-coated jicama into dry mixture, tossing to coat well.

4. Spray the Air Fryer basket with olive oil and add fries. Set temperature to 350°F, and set time to 5 minutes. Toss halfway into the cooking process.

Nutrition:

Calories 211

Fat 19g

Carbs 16g

Protein 9g

Lemon bell peppers

Preparation Time: 5 minutes

Cooking Time: 20 minutes

Servings: 4

Ingredients:

- 1 ½ lb. Mixed bell peppers; halved and deseeded
- 2 tbsp. Lemon juice
- 2 tbsp. Balsamic vinegar
- 2 tsp. Lemon zest, grated
- Parsley; chopped.

Directions:

1. Put the peppers in your Air Fryer's basket and cook at 350°f for 15 minutes.
2. Peel the bell peppers, mix them with the rest of the ingredients, toss and serve

Nutrition:

Calories 151

Fat 2g

Carbs 5g

Protein 5g

Cauliflower pizza crust

Preparation Time: 5 minutes

Cooking Time: 20 minutes

Servings: 6

Ingredients:

- 1(12-oz.) Steamer bag cauliflower
- 1 large egg.
- ½ cup shredded sharp cheddar cheese.
- 2 tbsp. Blanched finely ground almond flour
- 1 tsp. Italian blend seasoning

Directions:

1. Cook cauliflower according to package. Take out from bag and place into a paper towel to remove excess water. Place cauliflower into a large bowl.
2. Add almond flour, cheese, egg, and italian seasoning to the bowl and mix well

3. Cut a piece of parchment to fit your Air Fryer basket. Press cauliflower into 6-inch round circle. Place into the Air Fryer basket. Adjust the temperature to 360°F and set the timer for 11 minutes. After 7 minutes, flip the pizza crust
4. Add preferred toppings to pizza. Place back into Air Fryer basket and cook an additional 4 minutes or until fully cooked and golden. Serve immediately.

Nutrition:

Calories 230

Fat 14.2g

Carbs 10g

Protein 14.9g

Savoy cabbage and tomatoes

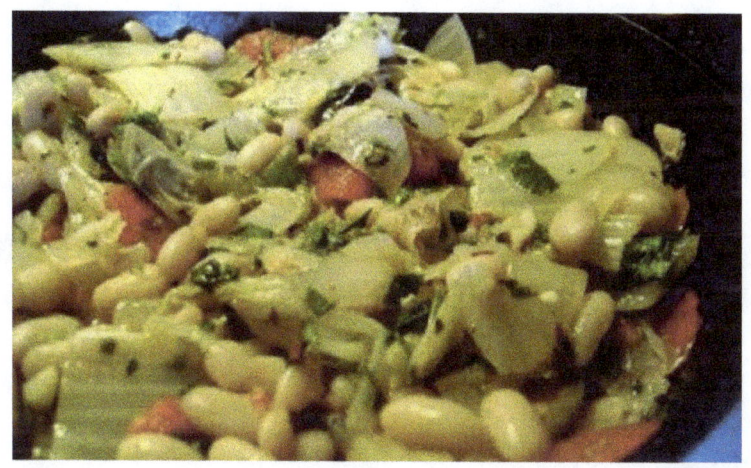

Preparation Time: 5 minutes

Cooking Time: 20 minutes

Servings: 4

Ingredients:

- 2 spring onions; chopped.
- 1 savoy cabbage, shredded
- 1 tbsp. Parsley; chopped.
- 2 tbsp. Tomato sauce

- Salt and black pepper to taste.

Directions:

1. In a pan that fits your Air Fryer, mix the cabbage the rest of the ingredients except the parsley, toss, put the pan in the fryer and cook at 360°f for 15 minutes
2. Divide between plates and serve with parsley sprinkled on top.

Nutrition:

Calories 163

Fat 4g

Carbs 6g

Protein 7g

Cauliflower steak

Preparation Time: 5 minutes

Cooking Time: 10 minutes

Servings: 4

Ingredients:

- 1 medium head cauliflower
- ¼ cup blue cheese crumbles
- ¼ cup hot sauce
- ¼ cup full-fat ranch dressing
- 2 tbsp. Salted butter; melted.

Directions:

1. Remove cauliflower leaves. Slice the head in ½-inch-thick slices.
2. In a small bowl, mix hot sauce and butter. Brush the mixture over the cauliflower.
3. Place each cauliflower steak into the Air Fryer, working in batches if necessary. Adjust the

temperature to 400°F and set the timer for 7 minutes
4. When cooked, edges will begin turning dark and caramelized. To serve, sprinkle steaks with crumbled blue cheese. Drizzle with ranch dressing.

Nutrition:

Calories 122

Fat 8.4g

Carbs 7.7g

Protein 4.9g

Tomato, avocado and green beans

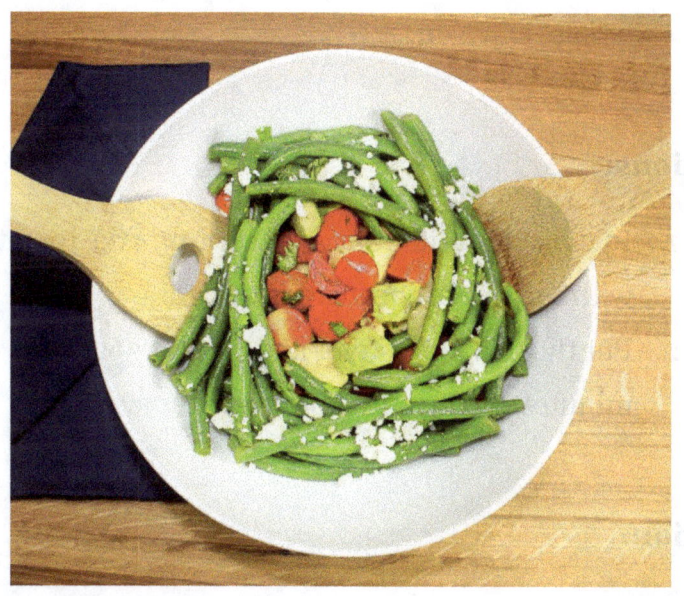

Preparation Time: 5 minutes

Cooking Time: 20 minutes

Servings: 4

Ingredients:

- ¼ lb. Green beans, trimmed and halved

- 1 avocado, peeled, pitted and cubed
- 1 pint mixed cherry tomatoes; halved
- 2 tbsp. Olive oil

Directions:

1. In a pan that fits your Air Fryer, mix the tomatoes with the rest of the ingredients, toss.
2. Put the pan in the fryer and cook at 360°F for 15 minutes. Transfer to bowls and serve

Nutrition:

Calories 151

Fat 3g

Carbs 4g

Protein 4g

Dill and garlic green beans

Preparation Time: 5 minutes

Cooking Time: 20 minutes

Servings: 4

Ingredients:

- 1 lb. Green beans, trimmed
- ½ cup bacon, cooked and chopped.
- 2 garlic cloves; minced
- 2 tbsp. Dill; chopped.
- Salt and black pepper to taste.

Directions:

1. In a pan that fits the Air Fryer, combine the green beans with the rest of the ingredients, toss.
2. Put the pan in the fryer and cook at 390°F for 15 minutes
3. Divide everything between plates and serve.

Nutrition:

Calories 180

Fat 3g

Carbs 4g

Protein 6g

Eggplant stacks

Preparation Time: 5 minutes

Cooking Time: 15 minutes

Servings: 4

Ingredients:

- 2 large tomatoes; cut into ¼-inch slices
- ¼ cup fresh basil, sliced
- 4oz. Fresh mozzarella; cut into ½-oz. Slices
- 1 medium eggplant; cut into ¼-inch slices
- 2 tbsp. Olive oil

Directions:

1. In a 6-inch round baking dish, place four slices of eggplant on the bottom. Put a slice of tomato on each eggplant round, then mozzarella, then eggplant. Repeat as necessary.

2. Drizzle with olive oil. Cover dish with foil and place dish into the Air Fryer basket. Adjust the temperature to 350°F and set the timer for 12 minutes.
3. When done, eggplant will be tender. Garnish with fresh basil to serve.

Nutrition:

Calories 195

Fat 12.7g

Carbs 12.7g

Protein 8.5g

Air Fried Spaghetti Squash

Preparation Time: 5 minutes

Cooking Time: 50 minutes

Servings: 4

Ingredients:

- ½ large spaghetti squash
- 2 tbsp. Salted butter; melted.
- 1 tbsp. Coconut oil
- 1 tsp. Dried parsley.
- ½ tsp. Garlic powder.

Directions:

1. Brush shell of spaghetti squash with coconut oil. Place the skin side down and brush the inside with butter. Sprinkle with garlic powder and parsley.
2. Place squash with the skin side down into the Air Fryer basket. Adjust the temperature to 350°F and set the timer for 30 minutes

3. When the timer beeps, flip the squash so skin side is up and cook an additional 15 minutes or until fork tender. Serve warm.

Nutrition:

Calories 182

Fat 11.7g

Carbs 18.2g

Protein 1.9g

Beets and Blue Cheese Salad

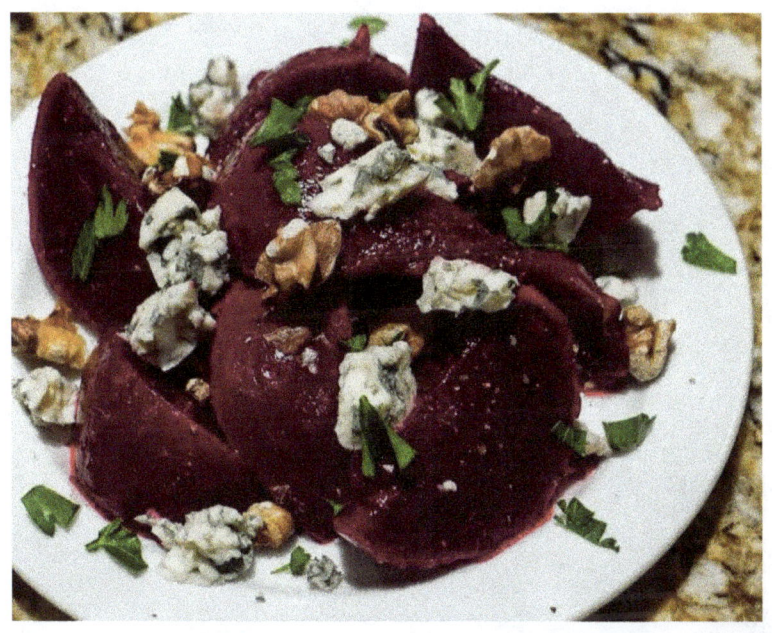

Preparation Time: 10 minutes

Cooking Time: 15 minutes

Servings: 6

Ingredients:

- 6 beets, peeled and quartered

- Salt and black pepper to the taste
- ¼ cup blue cheese, crumbled
- 1 tbsp. olive oil

Directions:

Put beets in your Air Fryer, cook them at 350°F for 14 minutes and transfer them to a bowl. Add blue cheese, salt, pepper and oil, toss and serve. Enjoy!

Nutrition:

Calories 100

Fat 4g

Carbs 10g

Protein 5g

Broccoli Salad

Preparation Time: 10 minutes

Cooking Time: 10 minutes

Servings: 4

Ingredients:

- 1 broccoli head, with separated florets
- 1 tbsp. peanut oil
- 6 cloves of garlic, minced
- 1 tbsp. Chinese rice wine vinegar
- Salt and black pepper to taste

Directions:

In a bowl, mix broccoli half of the oil with salt, pepper and, toss, transfer to your Air Fryer and cook at 350°F for 8 minutes. Halfway through, shake the fryer. Take the broccoli out and put it into a salad bowl, add the rest of the peanut oil, garlic and rice vinegar, mix really well and serve. Enjoy!

Nutrition:

Calories 121

Fat 3g

Carbs 4g

Protein 4g

Roasted Brussels Sprouts with Tomatoes

Preparation Time: 5 minutes

Cooking Time: 10 minutes

Servings: 4

Ingredients:

- 1-lb. Brussels sprouts, trimmed
- Salt and black pepper to the taste
- 6cherry tomatoes, halved
- ¼ cup green onions, chopped
- 1 tbsp. olive oil

Directions:

Season Brussels sprouts with salt and pepper, put them in your Air Fryer and cook at 350°F for 10 minutes. Transfer them to a bowl, add salt, pepper, cherry tomatoes, green onions and olive oil, toss well and serve. Enjoy!

Nutrition:

Calories 121

Fat 4g

Carbs 11g

Protein 4g

Cheesy Brussels Sprouts

Preparation Time: 10 minutes

Cooking Time: 10 minutes

Servings: 4

Ingredients:

- 1 lb. Brussels sprouts, washed
- Juice of 1 lemon
- Salt and black pepper to the taste
- 2 tbsp. butter
- 3 tbsp. parmesan, grated

Directions:

Put Brussels sprouts in your Air Fryer, cook them at 350°F for 8 minutes and transfer them to a bowl. Warm up a pan over moderate heat with the butter, then add lemon juice, salt and pepper, whisk well and add to Brussels sprouts. Add parmesan, toss until parmesan melts and serve. Enjoy!

Nutrition:

Calories 152

Fat 6g

Carbs 8g

Protein 12g

Sweet Baby Carrots Dish

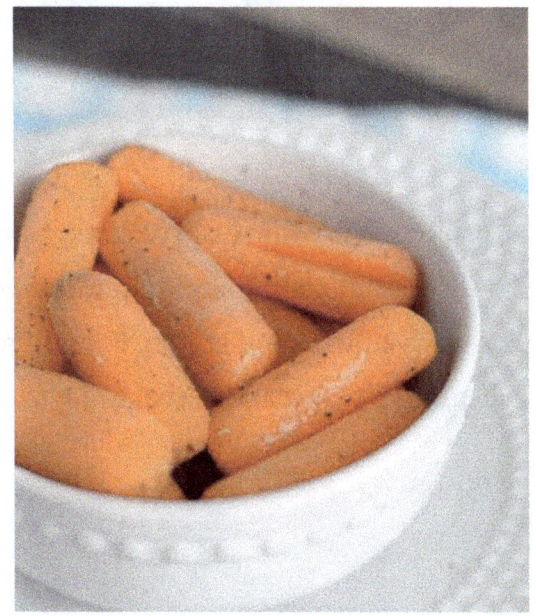

Preparation Time: 10 minutes

Cooking Time: 10 minutes

Servings: 4

Ingredients:

- 2 cups baby carrots

- A pinch of salt and black pepper
- 1 tbsp. brown sugar
- ½ tbsp. butter, melted

Directions:

In a dish that fits your Air Fryer, mix baby carrots with butter, salt, pepper and sugar, toss, introduce in your Air Fryer and cook at 350°F for 10 minutes. Divide among plates and serve. Enjoy!

Nutrition:

Calories 100

Fat 2g

Carbs 7g

Protein 4g

Seasoned Leeks

Preparation Time: 10 minutes

Cooking Time: 10 minutes

Servings: 4

Ingredients:

- 4leeks, washed, halved
- Salt and black pepper to taste
- 1 tbsp. butter, melted
- 1 tbsp. lemon juice

Directions:

Rub leeks with melted butter, season with salt and pepper, put in your Air Fryer and cook at 350°F for 7 minutes. Arrange on a platter, drizzle lemon juice all over and serve. Enjoy!

Nutrition:

Calories 100

Fat 4g

Carbs 6g

Protein 2g

Crispy Potatoes and Parsley

Preparation Time: 10 minutes

Cooking Time: 10 minutes

Servings: 4

Ingredients:

- 1-lb. gold potatoes, cut into wedges
- Salt and black pepper to the taste
- 2 tbsp. olive oil
- Juice from ½ lemon
- ¼ cup parsley leaves, chopped

Directions:

1. Rub potatoes with salt, pepper, lemon juice and olive oil, put them in your Air Fryer and cook at 350°F for 10 minutes. Divide among plates, sprinkle parsley on top and serve. Enjoy!

Nutrition:

Calories 152

Fat 3g

Carbs 17g

Protein 4g

Garlic Tomatoes

Preparation Time: 10 minutes

Cooking Time: 15 minutes

Servings: 4

Ingredients:

- 4 garlic cloves, crushed
- 1-lb. mixed cherry tomatoes
- 3 thyme springs, chopped
- Salt and black pepper to the taste
- ¼ cup olive oil

Directions:

In a bowl, mix tomatoes with salt, black pepper, garlic, olive oil and thyme, toss to coat, introduce in your Air Fryer and cook at 360°F for 15 minutes. Divide tomatoes mix on plates and serve. Enjoy!

Nutrition:

Calories 100

Fat 0g

Carbs 1g

Protein 6g

Easy Green Beans and Potatoes

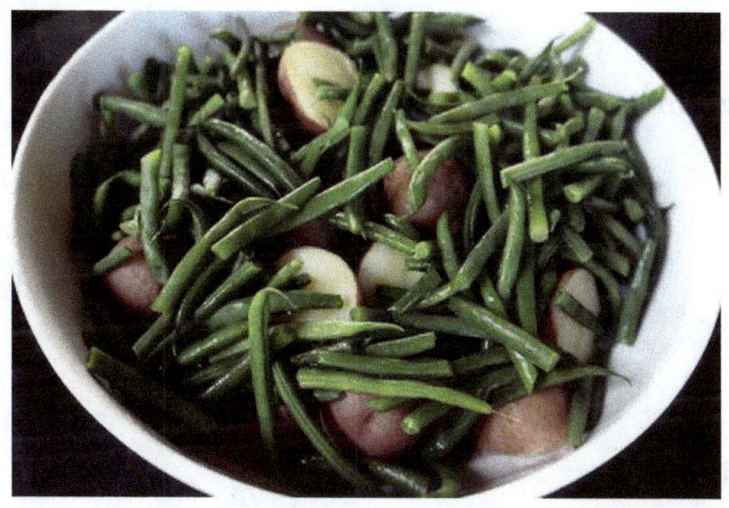

Preparation Time: 10 minutes

Cooking Time: 15 minutes

Servings: 5

Ingredients:

- 2 lb. green beans
- 6 new potatoes, halved
- Salt and black pepper to the taste

- A drizzle of olive oil
- 6 bacon slices, cooked and chopped

Directions:

In a bowl, mix green beans with potatoes, salt, pepper and oil, toss, transfer to your Air Fryer and cook at 390°F for 15 minutes. Divide among plates and serve with bacon sprinkled on top. Enjoy!

Nutrition:

Calories 374

Fat 15g

Carbs 28g

Protein 12g

Green Beans and Tomatoes

Preparation Time: 10 minutes

Cooking Time: 15 minutes

Servings: 4

Ingredients:

- 1 pint cherry tomatoes
- 1 lb. green beans
- 2 tbsp. olive oil
- Salt and black pepper to the taste

Directions:

In a bowl, mix cherry tomatoes with green beans, olive oil, salt and pepper, toss, transfer to your Air Fryer and cook at 400°F for 15 minutes. Divide among plates and serve right away. Enjoy!

Nutrition:

Calories 162

Fat 6g

Carbs 8g

Protein 9g

Flavored Asparagus

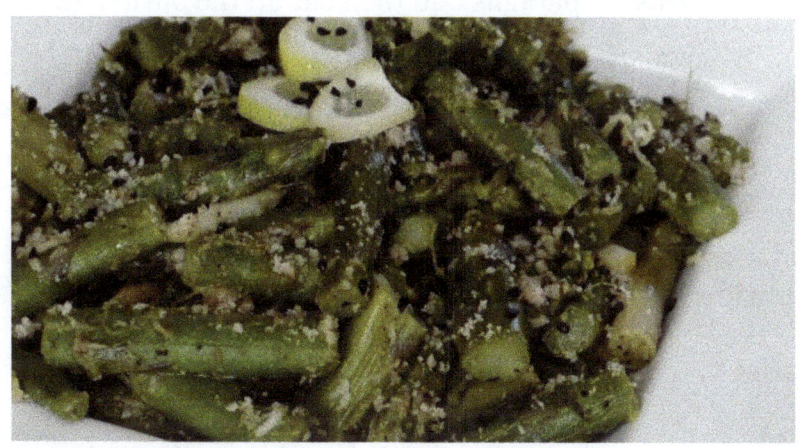

Preparation Time: 5 minutes

Cooking Time: 30 minutes

Servings: 2

Ingredients:

- Nutritional yeast
- Olive oil non-stick spray
- One bunch of asparagus

Directions:

- Wash asparagus and then cut off the bushy, woody ends. Drizzle asparagus with olive oil spray and sprinkle with yeast. In your Air Fryer, lay asparagus in a singular layer. Cook 8 minutes at 360°F.

Nutrition:

Calories 17

Fat 4g

Carbs 32g

Protein 24g

Spaghetti Squash Tots

Preparation Time: 5 minutes

Cooking Time: 15 minutes

Servings: 10

Ingredients:

- ¼ tsp. pepper
- ½ tsp. salt
- 1 thinly sliced scallion
- 1 spaghetti squash

Directions:

1. Wash and cut the squash in lengthwise. Scrape out the seeds. With a fork, remove spaghetti meat by strands and throw out skins. In a clean towel, toss in squash and wring out as much moisture as possible.
2. Place in a bowl and with a knife slice through meat a few times to cut up smaller. Add pepper, salt, and scallions to squash and mix well. Create "tot" shapes

with your hands and place in Air Fryer. Spray with olive oil. Cook 15 minutes at 350°F until golden and crispy!

Nutrition:

Calories 231

Fat 18g

Carbs 3g

Protein 5g

Cinnamon Butternut Squash Fries

Preparation Time: 10 minutes

Cooking Time: 10 minutes

Servings: 2

Ingredients:

- 1 pinch of salt
- 1 tbsp. powdered unprocessed sugar
- 2 tsp. cinnamon
- 1 tbsp. coconut oil
- 10 oz. pre-cut butternut squash fries

Directions:

In a plastic bag, pour in all ingredients. Coat fries with other components till coated and sugar is dissolved. Spread coated fries into a single layer in the Air Fryer. Cook 10 minutes at 390°F until crispy.

Nutrition:

Calories 175

Fat 8g

Carbs 3g

Protein 1g

Cheesy Roasted Sweet Potatoes

Preparation Time: 5 minutes

Cooking Time: 20 minutes

Servings: 4

Ingredients:

- 2 large sweet potatoes, peeled and sliced
- 1 tsp. olive oil
- 1 tbsp. white balsamic vinegar
- 1 tsp. dried thyme
- ¼ cup grated Parmesan cheese

Directions:

1. In a big bowl, shower the sweet potato slices with the olive oil and toss.
2. Sprinkle with the balsamic vinegar and thyme and toss again.
3. Sprinkle the potatoes with the Parmesan cheese and toss to coat.

4. Roast the slices, in batches, in the Air Fryer basket for 18 to 23 minutes at 375°F, tossing the sweet potato slices in the basket once during cooking, until tender.
5. Repeat with the remaining sweet potato slices. Serve immediately.

Nutrition:

Calories 100

Fat 3g

Carbs 15g

Protein 4g

Salty Lemon Artichokes

Preparation Time: 15 minutes

Cooking Time: 45 minutes

Servings: 2

Ingredients:

- 1 lemon
- 2 artichokes
- 1 tsp. kosher salt
- 1 garlic head
- 2 tsp. olive oil

Directions:

1. Cut off the edges of the artichokes.
2. Cut the lemon into halves.
3. Peel the garlic head and chop the garlic cloves roughly.
4. Then place the chopped garlic in the artichokes.
5. Sprinkle the artichokes with olive oil and kosher salt.

6. Then squeeze the lemon juice into the artichokes.
7. Wrap the artichokes in the foil.
8. Preheat the Air Fryer to 330°F.
9. Place the wrapped artichokes in the Air Fryer and cook for 45 minutes.
10. When the artichokes are cooked – discard the foil and serve.

Nutrition:

Calories 133

Fat 5g

Carbs 21.7g

Protein 6g

Asparagus & Parmesan

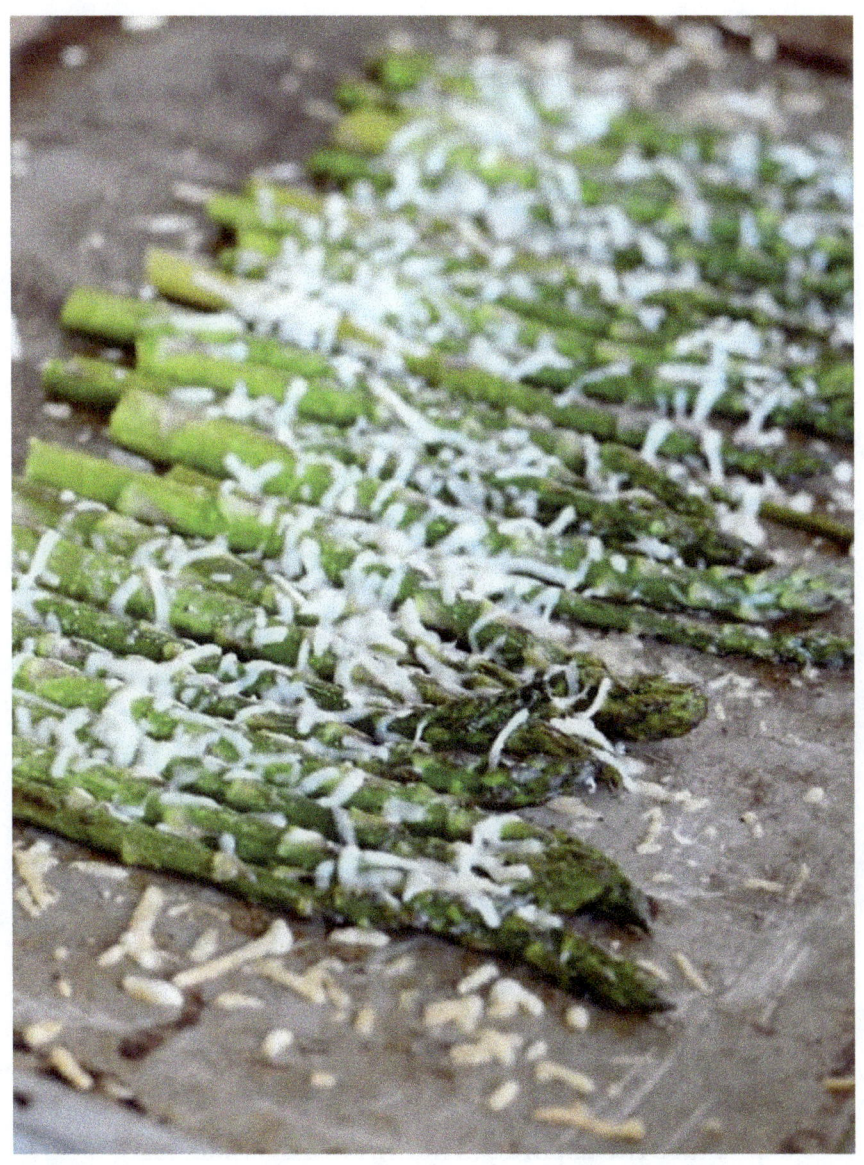

Preparation Time: 10 minutes

Cooking Time: 6 minutes

Servings: 2

Ingredients:

- 1 tsp. sesame oil
- 11 oz asparagus
- 1 tsp. chicken stock
- ½ tsp. ground white pepper
- 3 oz Parmesan

Directions:

1. Wash the asparagus and chop it roughly.
2. Sprinkle the chopped asparagus with the chicken stock and ground white pepper.
3. Then sprinkle the vegetables with the sesame oil and shake them.
4. Place the asparagus in the Air Fryer basket.
5. Cook the vegetables for 4 minutes at 400°F.
6. Meanwhile, shred Parmesan cheese.

7. When the time is over – shake the asparagus gently and sprinkle with the shredded cheese.
8. Cook the asparagus for 2 minutes more at 400°F.
9. After this, transfer the cooked asparagus in the serving plates.
10. Serve and taste it!

Nutrition:

Calories 189

Fat 11.6g

Carbs 7.9g

Protein 17.2g

Corn on Cobs

Preparation Time: 10 minutes

Cooking Time: 10 minutes

Servings: 2

Ingredients:

- 2 fresh corn on cobs
- 2 tsp. butter
- 1 tsp. salt
- 1 tsp. paprika
- ¼ tsp. olive oil

Directions:

1. Preheat the Air Fryer to 400°F.
2. Rub the corn on cobs with the salt and paprika.
3. Then sprinkle the corn on cobs with the olive oil.
4. Place the corn on cobs in the Air Fryer basket.
5. Cook the corn on cobs for 10 minutes.

6. When the time is over – transfer the corn on cobs in the serving plates and rub with the butter gently.
7. Serve the meal immediately.

Nutrition:

Calories 122

Fat 5.5g

Carbs 17.6g

Protein 3.2g

Onion Green Beans

Preparation Time: 10 minutes

Cooking Time: 12 minutes

Servings: 2

Ingredients:

- 11 oz green beans
- 1 tbsp. onion powder
- 1 tbsp. olive oil
- ½ tsp. salt
- ¼ tsp. chili flakes

Directions:

1. Wash the green beans carefully and place them in the bowl.
2. Sprinkle the green beans with the onion powder, salt, chili flakes, and olive oil.
3. Shake the green beans carefully.
4. Preheat the Air Fryer to 400°F.

5. Put the green beans in the Air Fryer and cook for 8 minutes.
6. After this, shake the green beans and cook them for 4 minutes more at 400°F.
7. When the time is over – shake the green beans.
8. Serve the side dish and enjoy!

Nutrition:

Calories 145

Fat 7.2g

Carbs 13.9g

Protein 3.2g

Dill Mashed Potato

Preparation Time: 10 minutes

Cooking Time: 15 minutes

Servings: 2

Ingredients:

- 2 potatoes
- 2 tbsp. fresh dill, chopped
- 1 tsp. butter
- ½ tsp. salt
- ¼ cup half and half

Directions:

1. Preheat the Air Fryer to 390°F.
2. Rinse the potatoes thoroughly and place them in the Air Fryer.
3. Cook the potatoes for 15 minutes.
4. After this, remove the potatoes from the Air Fryer.
5. Peel the potatoes.

6. Mash the potatoes with the help of the fork well.
7. Then add chopped fresh dill and salt.
8. Stir it gently and add butter and half and half.
9. Take the hand blender and blend the mixture well.
10. When the mashed potato is cooked – serve it immediately. Enjoy!

Nutrition:

Calories 211

Fat 5.7g

Carbs 36.5g

Protein 5.1g

Cream Potato

Preparation Time: 15 minutes

Cooking Time: 20 minutes

Servings: 2

Ingredients:

- 3 medium potatoes, scrubbed
- ½ tsp. kosher salt
- 1 tbsp. Italian seasoning
- 1/3 cup cream
- ½ tsp. ground black pepper

Directions:

1. Slice the potatoes.
2. Preheat the Air Fryer to 365°F.
3. Make the layer from the sliced potato in the Air Fryer basket.
4. Sprinkle the potato layer with the kosher salt and ground black pepper.

5. After this, make the second layer of the potato and sprinkle it with Italian seasoning.
6. Make the last layer of the sliced potato and pour the cream.
7. Cook the scallop potato for 20 minutes.
8. When the scalloped potato is cooked – let it chill to room temperature. Enjoy!

Nutrition:

Calories 269

Fat 4.7g

Carbs 52.6g

Protein 5.8g

Chard with Cheddar

Preparation Time: 10 minutes

Cooking Time: 11 minutes

Servings: 2

Ingredients:

- 3 oz Cheddar cheese, grated
- 10 oz Swiss chard
- 3 tbsp. cream
- 1 tbsp. sesame oil
- Salt and pepper to taste

Directions:

1. Wash Swiss chard carefully and chop it roughly.
2. After this, sprinkle chopped Swiss chard with the salt and ground white pepper.
3. Stir it carefully.
4. Sprinkle Swiss chard with the sesame oil and stir it carefully with the help of 2 spatulas.

5. Preheat the Air Fryer to 260°F.
6. Put chopped Swiss chard in the Air Fryer basket and cook for 6 minutes.
7. Shake it after 3 minutes of cooking.
8. Then pour the cream into the Air Fryer basket and mix it up.
9. Cook the meal for 3 minutes more.
10. Then increase the temperature to 400°F.
11. Sprinkle the meal with the grated cheese and cook for 2 minutes more.
12. After this, transfer the meal in the serving plates. Enjoy!

Nutrition:

Calories 272

Fat 22.3g

Carbs 6.7g

Protein 13.3g

Chili Squash Wedges

Preparation Time: 10 minutes

Cooking Time: 18 minutes

Servings: 2

Ingredients:

- 11 oz Acorn squash
- ½ tsp. salt
- tbsp. olive oil
- ½ tsp. chili pepper
- ½ tsp. paprika

Directions:

1. Cut Acorn squash into the serving wedges.
2. Sprinkle the wedges with salt, olive oil, chili pepper, and paprika.
3. Massage the wedges gently.
4. Preheat the Air Fryer to 400°F.

5. Put Acorn squash wedges in the Air Fryer basket and cook for 18 minutes.
6. Flip the wedges into another side after 9 minutes of cooking.
7. Serve the cooked meal hot. Enjoy!

Nutrition:

Calories 125

Fat 7.2g

Carbs 16.7g

Protein 1.4g

Honey Carrots with Greens

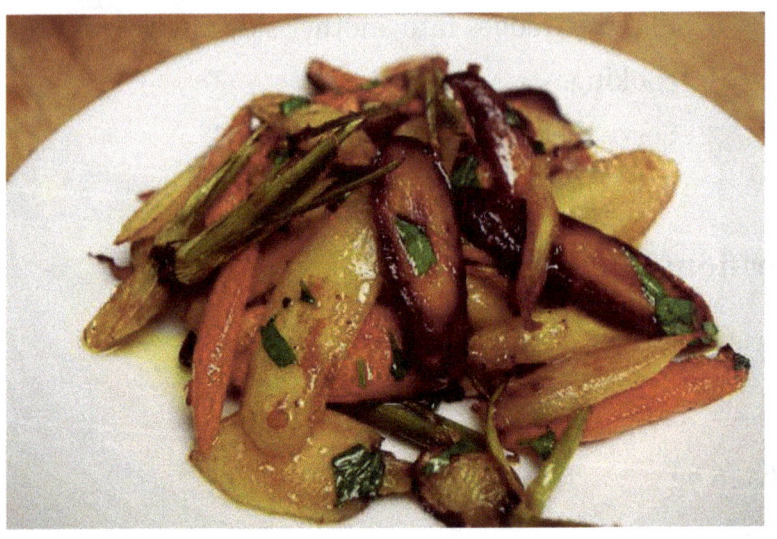

Preparation Time: 7 minutes

Cooking Time: 12 minutes

Servings: 2

Ingredients:

- 1 cup baby carrot
- ½ tsp. salt
- ½ tsp. white pepper

- 1 tbsp. honey
- 1 tsp. sesame oil

Directions:

1. Preheat the Air Fryer to 385°F.
2. Combine the baby carrot with salt, white pepper, and sesame oil.
3. Shake the baby carrot and transfer in the Air Fryer basket.
4. Cook the vegetables for 10 minutes.
5. After this, add honey and shake the vegetables.
6. Cook the meal for 2 minutes.
7. After this, shake the vegetables and serve immediately.

Nutrition:

Calories 83

Fat 2.4g

Carbs 16g

Protein 0.6g

South Asian Cauliflower Fritters

Preparation Time: 5 minutes

Cooking Time: 20 minutes

Servings: 4

Ingredients:

- 1 large chopped into florets cauliflower
- 3 tbsp. of Greek yogurt
- 3 tbsp. of flour
- ½ tsp. of ground turmeric
- ½ tsp. of ground cumin
- ½ tsp. of ground paprika
- 12 tsp. of ground coriander
- ½ tsp. of salt
- ½ tsp. of black pepper

Directions:

1. Using a large bowl, add and mix the Greek yogurt, flour, and seasonings properly.
2. Add the cauliflower florets and toss it until it is well covered
3. Heat up your Air Fryer to 390°F.
4. Grease your Air Fryer basket with a nonstick cooking spray and add half of the cauliflower florets to it.
5. Cook it for 10 minutes or until it turns golden brown and crispy, then shake it after 5 minutes. (Repeat this with the other half).
6. Serve and enjoy!

Nutrition:

Calories 120

Fat 4g

Carbs 14g

Protein 7.5g

Supreme Air-Fried Tofu

Preparation Time: 5 minutes

Cooking Time: 50 minutes

Servings: 4

Ingredients:

- 1 block of pressed and sliced into 1-inch cubes of extra-firm tofu
- 2 tbsp. of soy sauce
- 1 tsp. of seasoned rice vinegar
- 2 tsp.s of toasted sesame oil
- 1 tbsp. of cornstarch

Directions:

1. Using a bowl, add and toss the tofu, soy sauce, seasoned rice vinegar, sesame oil until it is properly covered.
2. Place it inside your refrigerator and allow to marinate for 30 minutes.

3. Preheat your Air Fryer to 370°F.
4. Add the cornstarch to the tofu mixture and toss it until it is properly covered.
5. Grease your Air Fryer basket with a nonstick cooking spray and add the tofu inside your basket.
6. Cook it for 20 minutes at 370°F, and shake it after 10 minutes.
7. Serve and enjoy!

Nutrition:

Calories 80

Fat 5.8g

Carbs 3g

Protein 5g

Lemon Bars

Preparation Time: 10 minutes

Cooking Time: 35 minutes

Servings: 8

Ingredients:

- ½ cup butter, melted
- 1 cup erythritol
- 1 and ¾ cups almond flour
- 3 eggs, whisked
- Juice of 3 lemons

Directions:

1. In a bowl, mix 1 cup flour with half of the erythritol and the butter, stir well and press into a baking dish that fits the Air Fryer lined with parchment paper.
2. Put the dish in your Air Fryer and cook at 350°F for 10 minutes.
3. In the meantime, in a bowl, blend the rest of the flour with the remaining erythritol and the other ingredients and whisk well.

4. Spread this over the crust, put the dish in the Air Fryer once more and cook at 350°F for 25 minutes.
5. Cool down, cut into bars and serve.

Nutrition:

Calories 210

Fat 12g

Carbs 4g

Protein 8g

Coconut Donuts

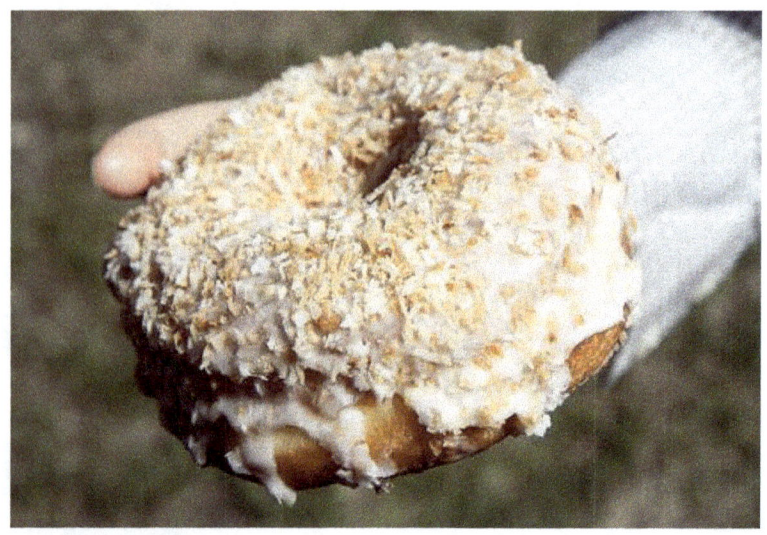

Preparation Time: 5 minutes

Cooking Time: 15 minutes

Servings: 4

Ingredients:

- 8 oz. coconut flour
- 1 egg, whisked
- and ½ tbsp. butter, melted

- 40 unces coconut milk
- 1 tsp. baking powder

Directions:

1. In a bowl, put all of the ingredients and mix well.
2. Shape donuts from this mix, place them in your Air Fryer's basket and cook at 370°F for 15 minutes. Serve warm.

Nutrition:

Calories 190

Fat 12g

Protein 6g

Carbs 4g

Blueberry Cream

Preparation Time: 4 minutes

Cooking Time: 20 minutes

Servings: 6

Ingredients:

- 2 cups blueberries
- Juice of ½ lemon
- 2 tbsp. water
- 1 tsp. vanilla extract
- 2 tbsp. swerve

Directions:

1. In a large bowl, put all ingredients and mix well.
2. Divide this into 6 ramekins, put them in the Air Fryer and cook at 340°F for 20 minutes
3. Cool down and serve.

Nutrition:

Calories 123
Fat 2g
Carbs 4g
Protein 3g

Blackberry Chia Jam

Preparation Time: 10 minutes

Cooking Time: 30 minutes

Servings: 12

Ingredients:

- 3cups blackberries
- ¼ cup swerve
- 4tbsp. lemon juice
- 4tbsp. chia seeds

Directions:

1. In a pan that suits the Air Fryer, combine all the ingredients: and toss.
2. Put the pan in the fryer and cook at 300°F for 30 minutes.
3. Divide into cups and serve cold.

Nutrition:
Calories 100
Fat 2g
Carbs 3g
Protein 1g

Mixed Berries Cream

Preparation Time: 5 minutes

Cooking Time: 30 minutes

Servings: 6

Ingredients:

- 12 oz. blackberries
- 6 oz. raspberries
- 12 oz. blueberries
- ¾ cup swerve
- 2 oz. coconut cream

Directions:
1. In a bowl, put all the ingredients: and mix well.
2. Divide this into 6 ramekins, put them in your Air Fryer and cook at 320°F for 30 minutes.
3. Cool down and serve it.

Nutrition:

Calories 100

Fat 1g

Carbs 2g

Protein 2g

Apple Chips

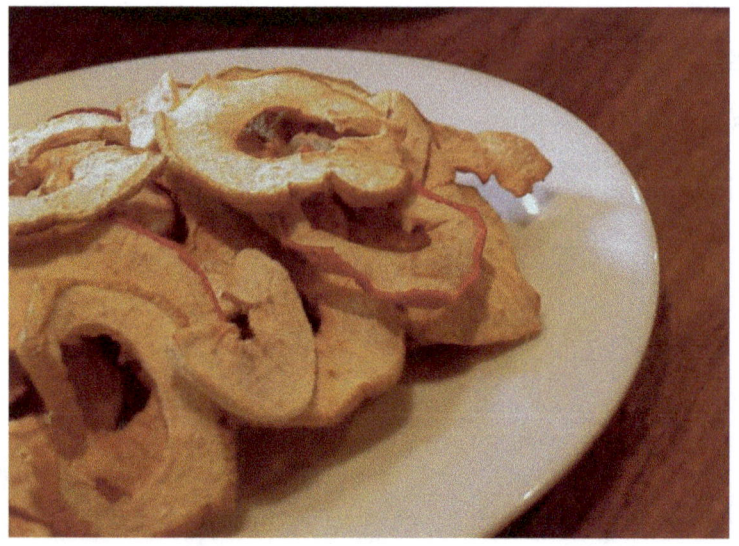

Preparation Time: 10 minutes

Cooking Time: 20 minutes

Servings: 2

Ingredients:

- 1 apple, sliced thinly
- Salt to taste

- ¼ tsp. ground cinnamon

Directions:

1. Preheat the Air Fryer to 350°F.
2. Toss the apple slices in salt and cinnamon.
3. Add to the Air Fryer. Cook for 20 minutes
4. Let cool before serving.

Nutrition:

Calories 59

Fat 0.2g

Carbs 15.6g

Protein 0.3g

Sweetened Plantains

Preparation Time: 5 minutes

Cooking Time: 8 minutes

Servings: 4

Ingredients:

- 2 ripe plantains, sliced
- 2 tsp.s avocado oil
- Salt to taste
- Maple syrup

Directions:

1. Toss the plantains in oil.
2. Season with salt.
3. Cook in the Air Fryer basket at 400°F for 10 minutes, shaking after 5 minutes.
4. Drizzle with maple syrup before serving.

Nutrition:

Calories 125

Fat 0.6g

Carbs 32g

Protein 1.2g

Roasted Bananas

Preparation Time: 5 minutes

Cooking Time: 5 minutes

Servings: 2

Ingredients:

- 2 cups bananas, cubed
- 1 tsp. avocado oil
- 1 tbsp. maple syrup
- 1 tsp. brown sugar
- 1 cup almond milk

Directions:

1. Coat the banana cubes with oil and maple syrup.
2. Sprinkle with brown sugar.
3. Cook at 375°F in the Air Fryer for 5 minutes.
4. Drizzle milk on top of the bananas before serving.

Nutrition:

Calories 107

Fat 0.7g

Carbs 27g

Protein 1.3g

Pear Crisp

Preparation Time: 10 minutes

Cooking Time: 25 minutes

Servings: 2

Ingredients:

- 1 cup flour
- 1 stick vegan butter
- 1 tbsp. cinnamon
- ½ cup sugar
- 2 pears, cubed

Directions:

1. Mix flour and butter to form crumbly texture.
2. Add cinnamon and sugar.
3. Put the pears in the Air Fryer.
4. Pour and spread the mixture on top of the pears.
5. Cook at 350°F for 25 minutes.

Nutrition:

Calories 544

Fat 0.9g

Carbs 132.3g

Protein 7.4g

www.ingramcontent.com/pod-product-compliance
Lightning Source LLC
Chambersburg PA
CBHW070734030426
42336CB00013B/1970